This Book Belongs to

____

____

____

Note: if using real makeup, allow page to dry completely before turning or closing. A short burst from a hair dryer can aid this process.

Inspiration Board

Color Palettes & Patterns

Masks

Beads & Bling

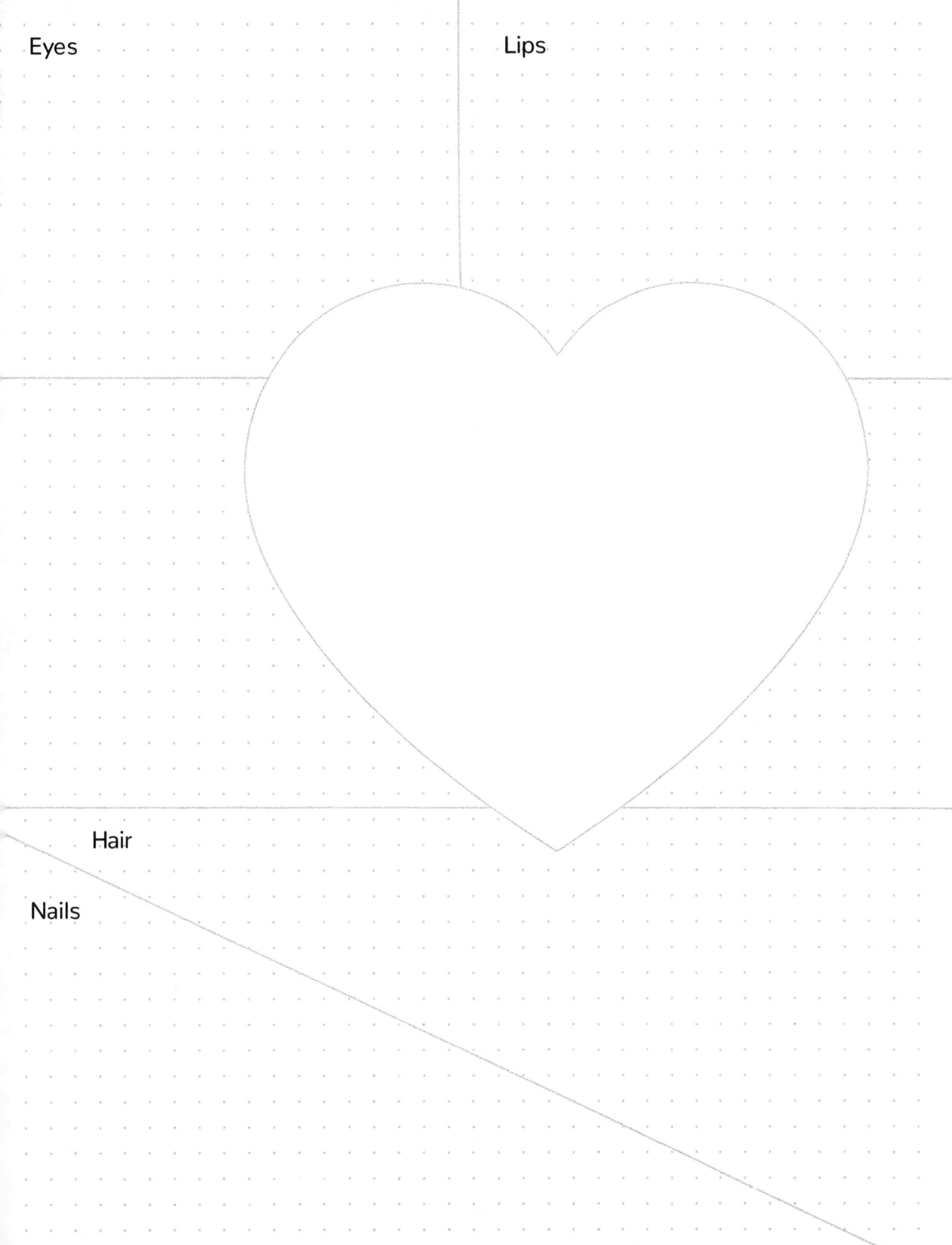
Eyes
Lips
Hair
Nails

Name of Look _________________________   **Evening** ◯   **Daytime** ◯

Theme ____

Face

Moisturizer

____

Concealer

____

Foundation

____

Highlight/Blush

____

Eyes

Brows

____

Eyelid

____

Liner

____

Crease

____

Mascara

____

Lips

Liner

____

Lip Color

____

Gloss

____

Notes

Makeup

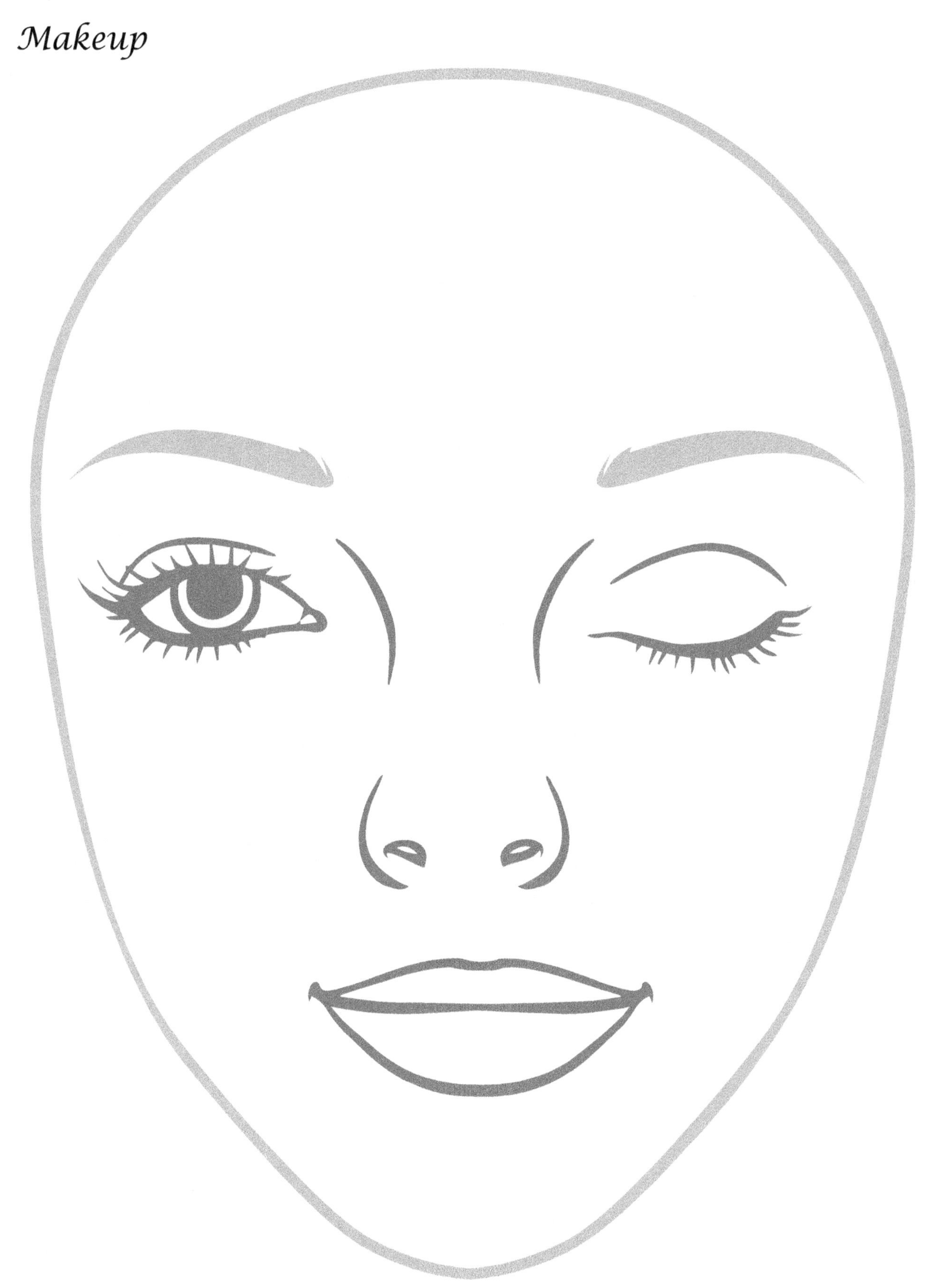

Name of Look _______________________________ **Evening** ◯ **Daytime** ◯

Theme ____

Face

Moisturizer

____

Concealer

____

Foundation

____

Highlight/Blush

____

Eyes

Brows

____

Eyelid

____

Liner

____

Crease

____

Mascara

____

Lips

Liner

____

Lip Color

____

Gloss

____

____

Notes

Makeup

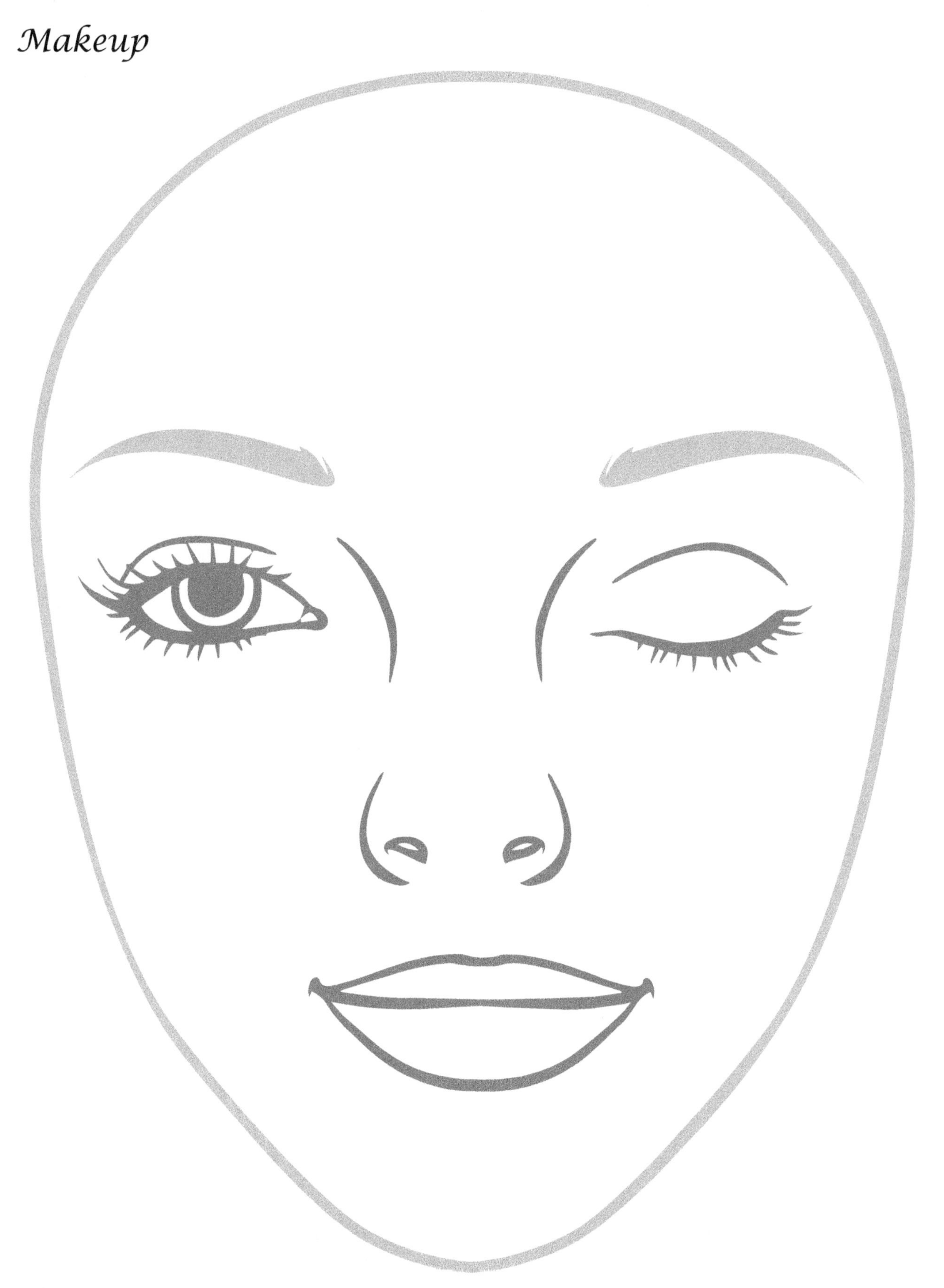

Name of Look _______________________________   Evening ○   Daytime ○

Theme ____

Face

Moisturizer

Concealer

Foundation

Highlight/Blush

Eyes

Brows

Eyelid

Liner

Crease

Mascara

Lips

Liner

Lip Color

Gloss

Notes

Makeup

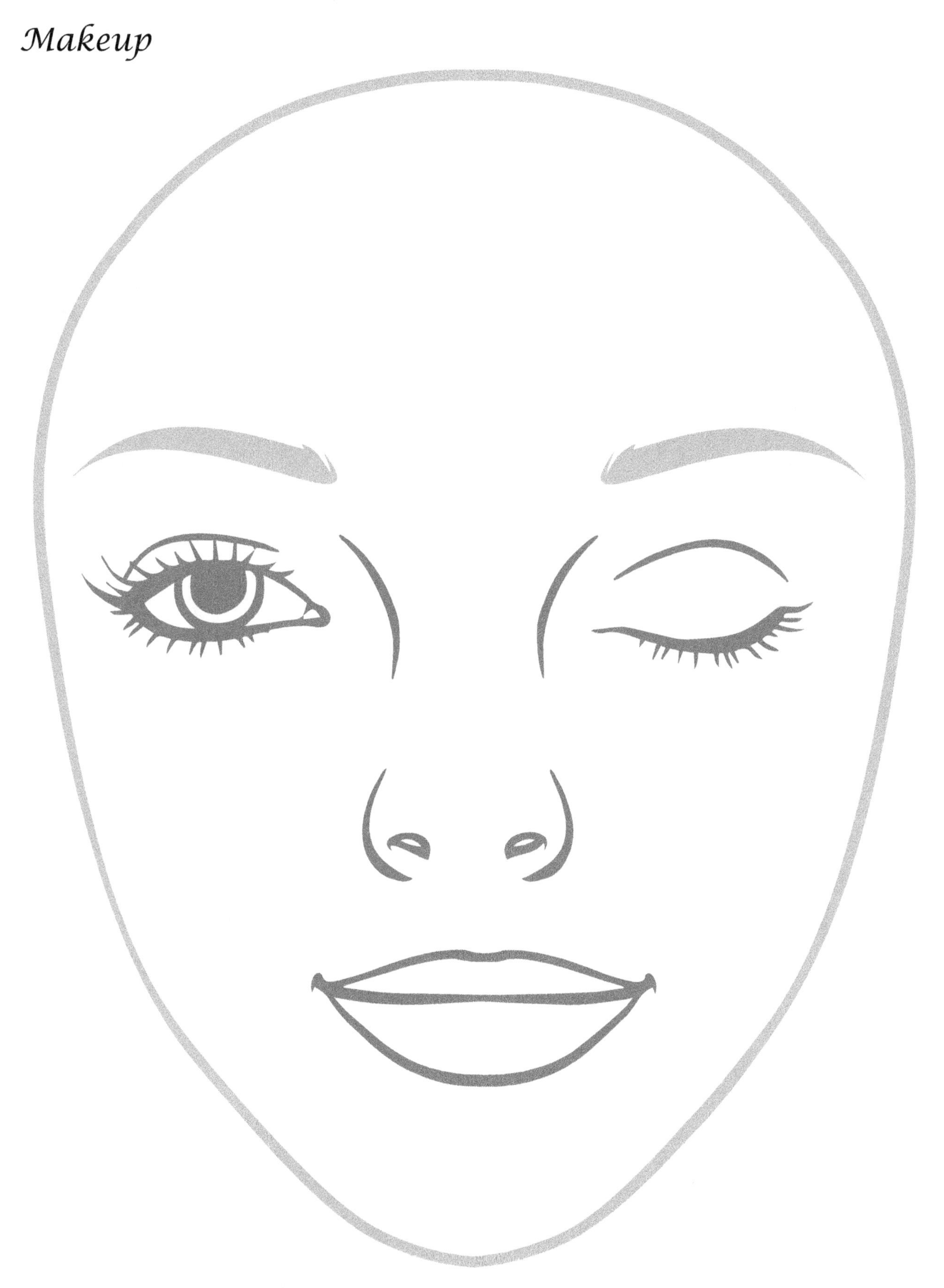

Name of Look _______________________   Evening ◯   Daytime ◯

Theme ____

Face

Moisturizer

____

Concealer

____

Foundation

____

Highlight/Blush

____

Eyes

Brows

____

Eyelid

____

Liner

____

Crease

____

Mascara

____

Lips

Liner

____

Lip Color

____

Gloss

____

Notes

Makeup

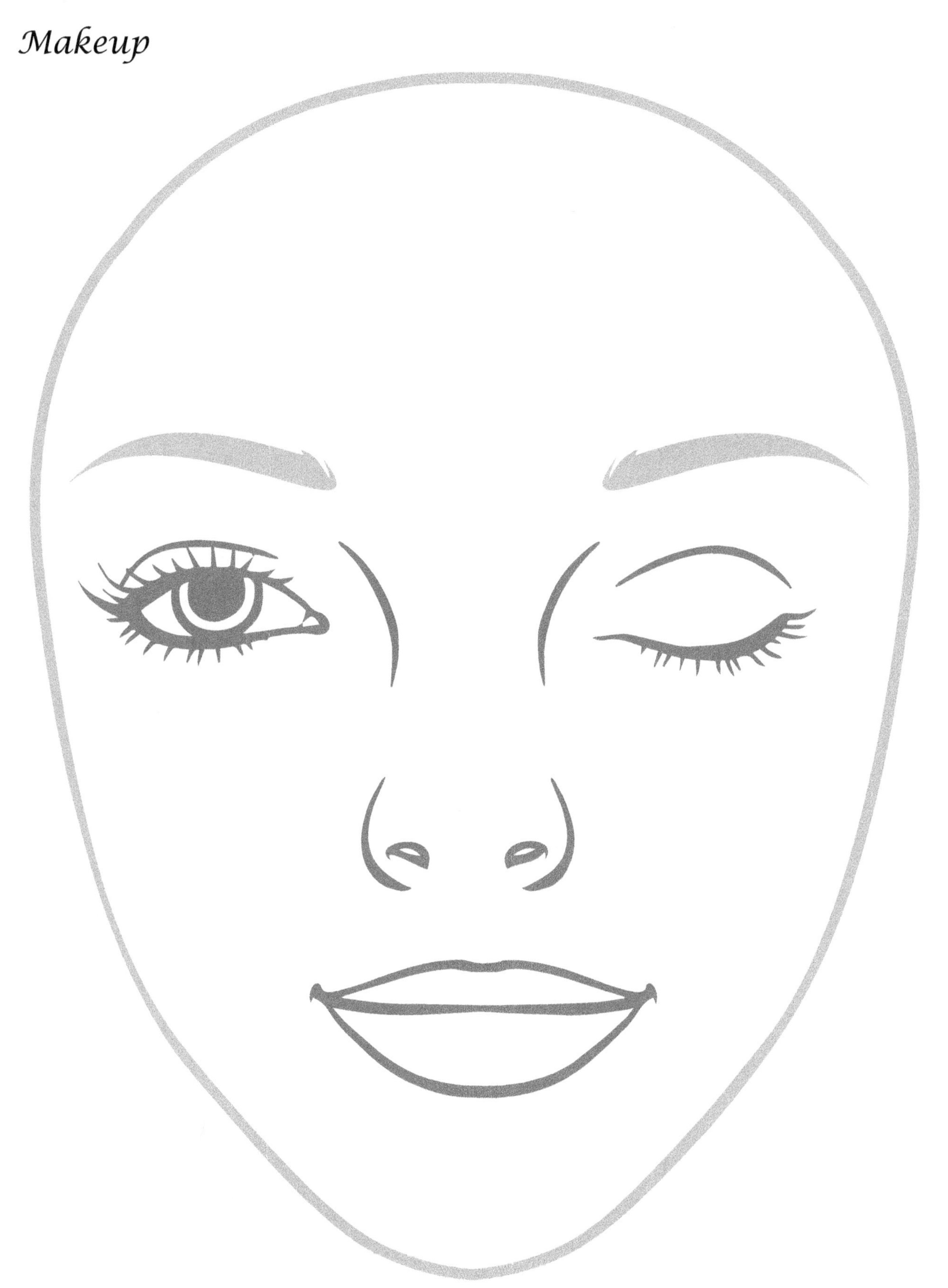

Inspiration Board

Color Palettes & Patterns

Masks

Beads & Bling

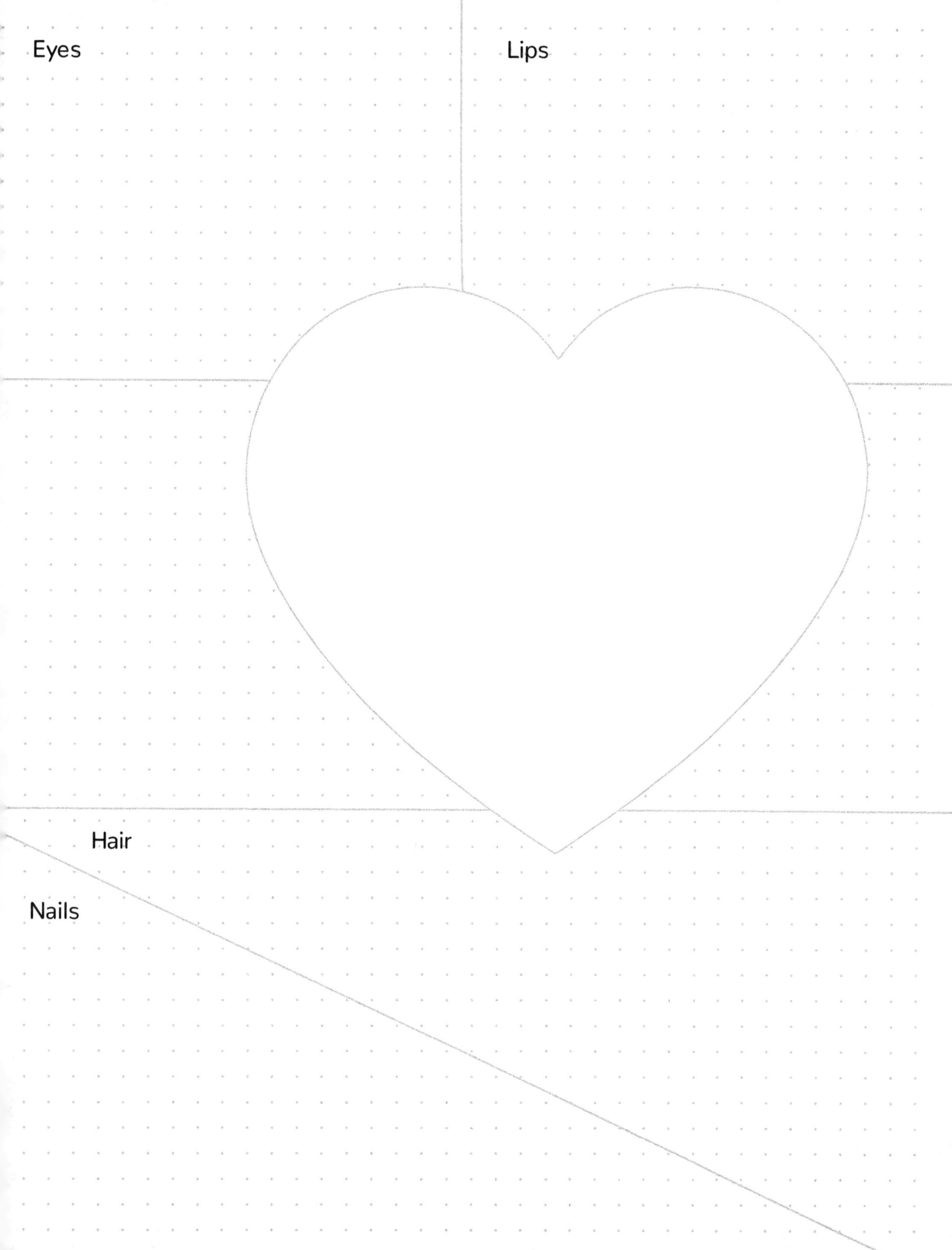Eyes
Lips
Hair
Nails

Name of Look _______________________   **Evening** ◯   **Daytime** ◯

Theme _______________________________________

Face	**Eyes**	**Lips**
Moisturizer	Brows	Liner
Concealer	Eyelid	Lip Color
Foundation	Liner	Gloss
Highlight/Blush	Crease	
	Mascara	

Notes

Makeup

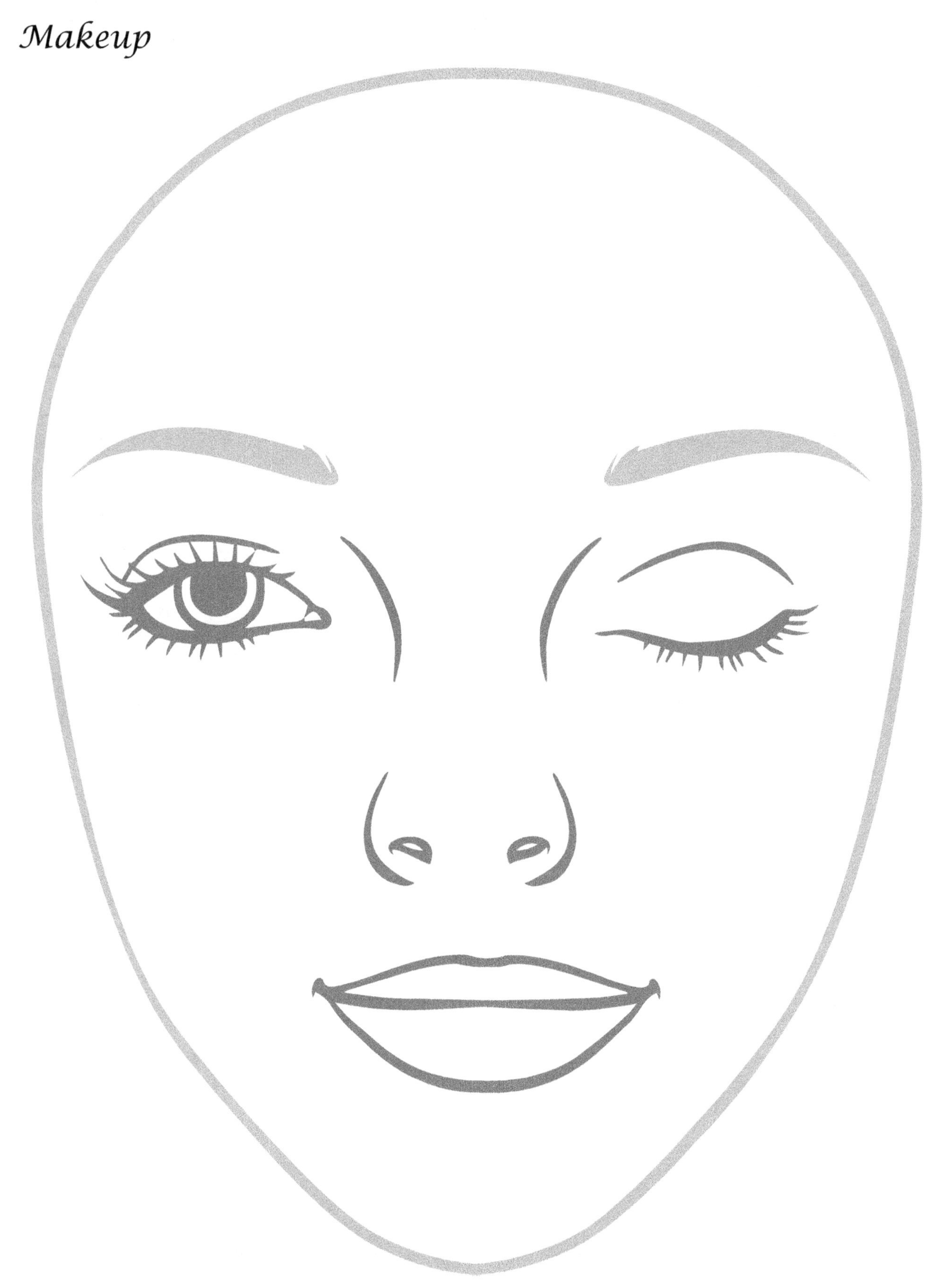

Name of Look ___________________________   **Evening** ◯   **Daytime** ◯

Theme ___________________________

Face	**Eyes**	**Lips**
Moisturizer	Brows	Liner
Concealer	Eyelid	Lip Color
Foundation	Liner	Gloss
Highlight/Blush	Crease	
	Mascara	

Notes

Makeup

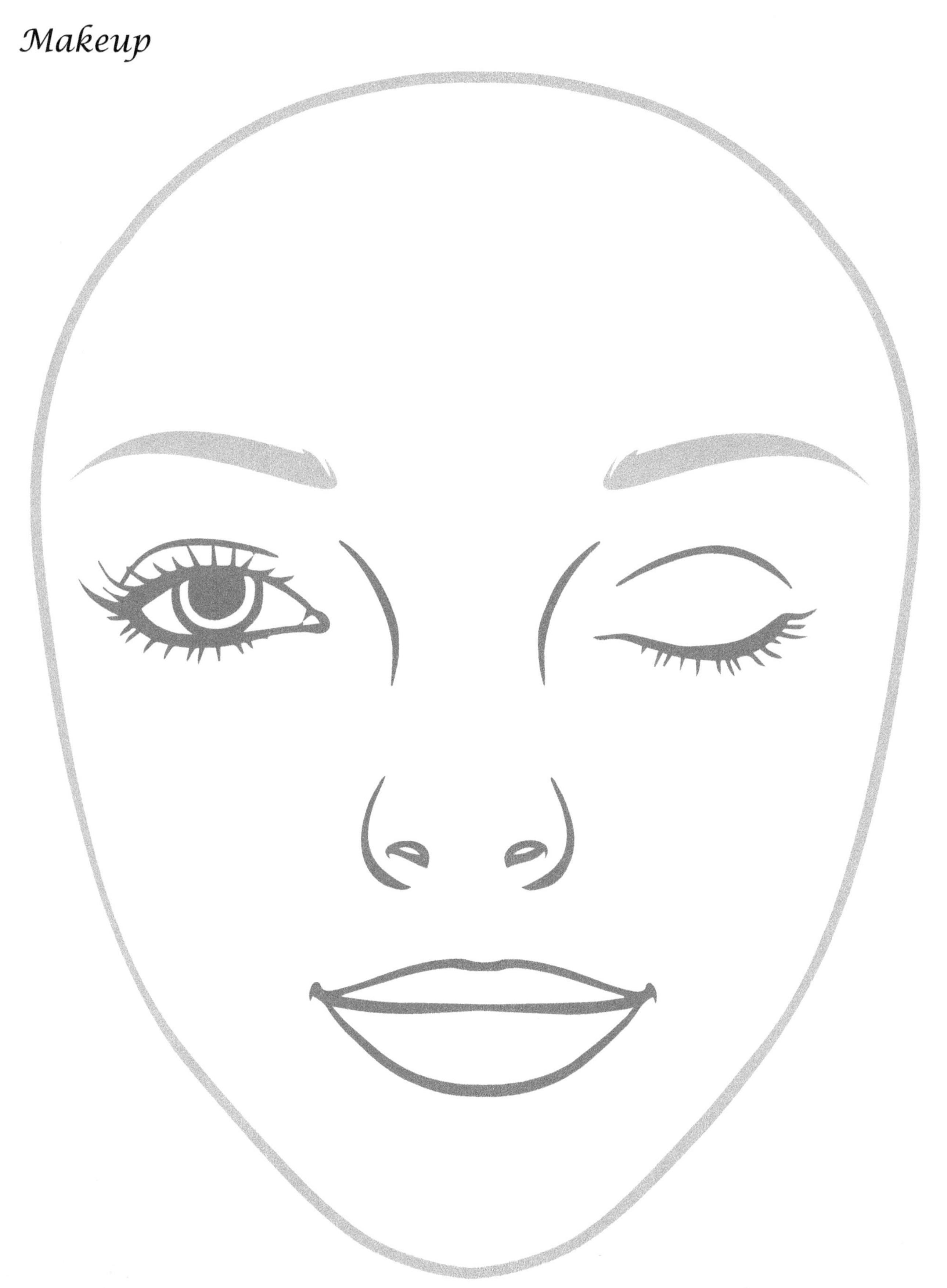

Name of Look ___________________________   Evening ◯   Daytime ◯

Theme ____

Face

Moisturizer

____

Concealer

____

Foundation

____

Highlight/Blush

____

Eyes

Brows

____

Eyelid

____

Liner

____

Crease

____

Mascara

____

Lips

Liner

____

Lip Color

____

Gloss

____

____

____

Notes

Makeup

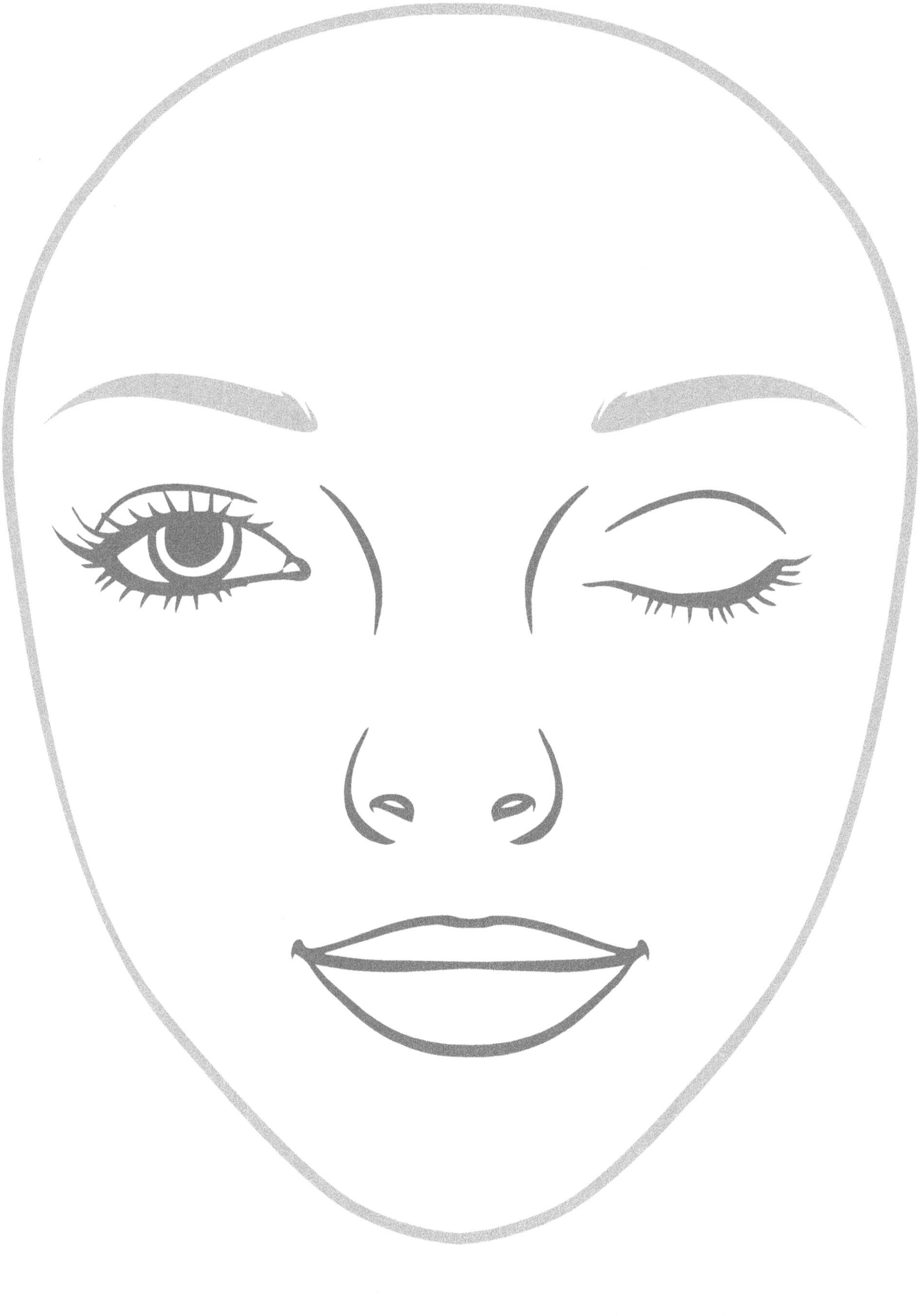

Name of Look Evening ◯   **Daytime** ◯

Theme

Face

Moisturizer

Concealer

Foundation

Highlight/Blush

Eyes

Brows

Eyelid

Liner

Crease

Mascara

Lips

Liner

Lip Color

Gloss

Notes

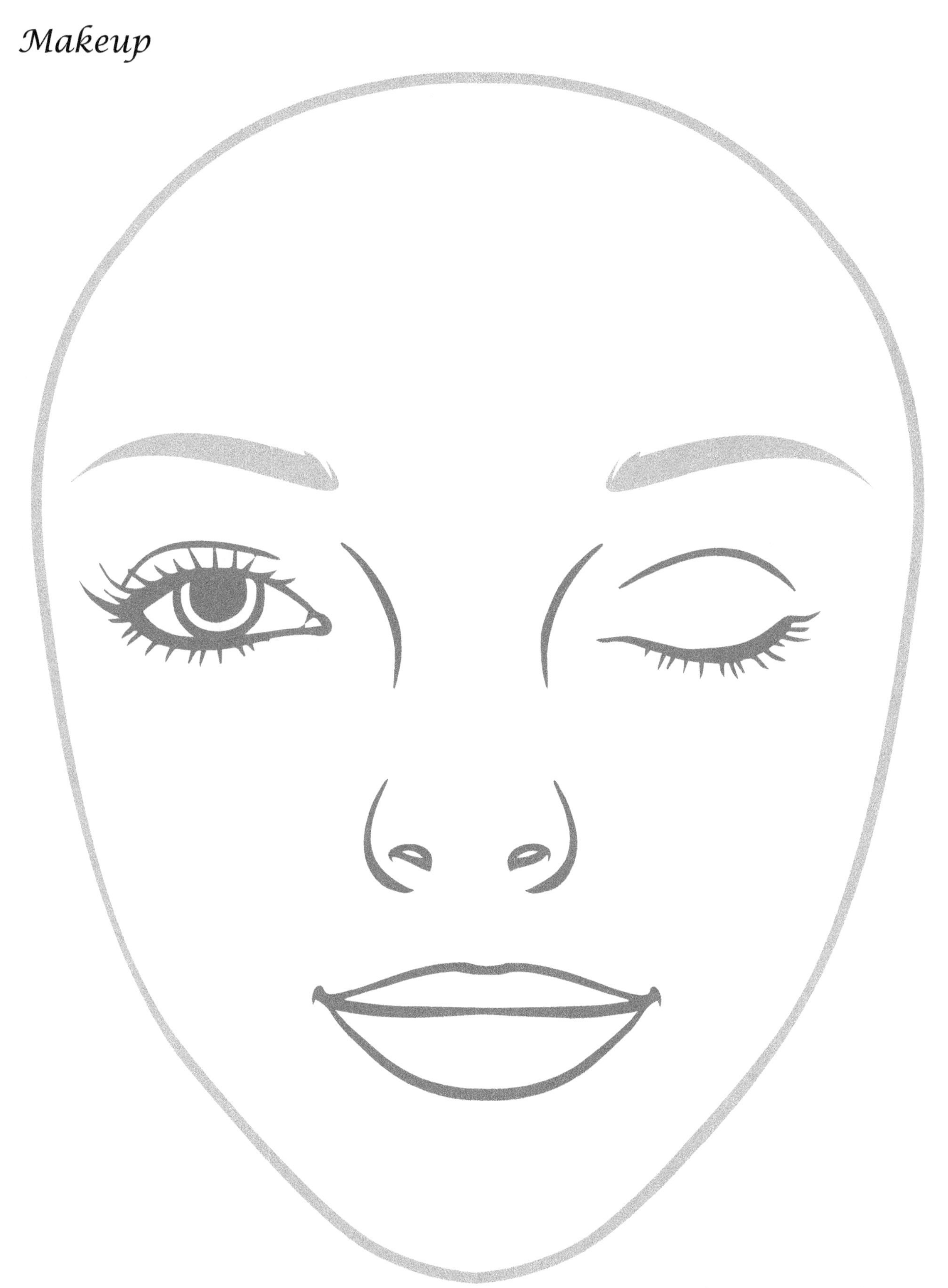

Inspiration Board

Color Palettes & Patterns

Masks

Beads & Bling

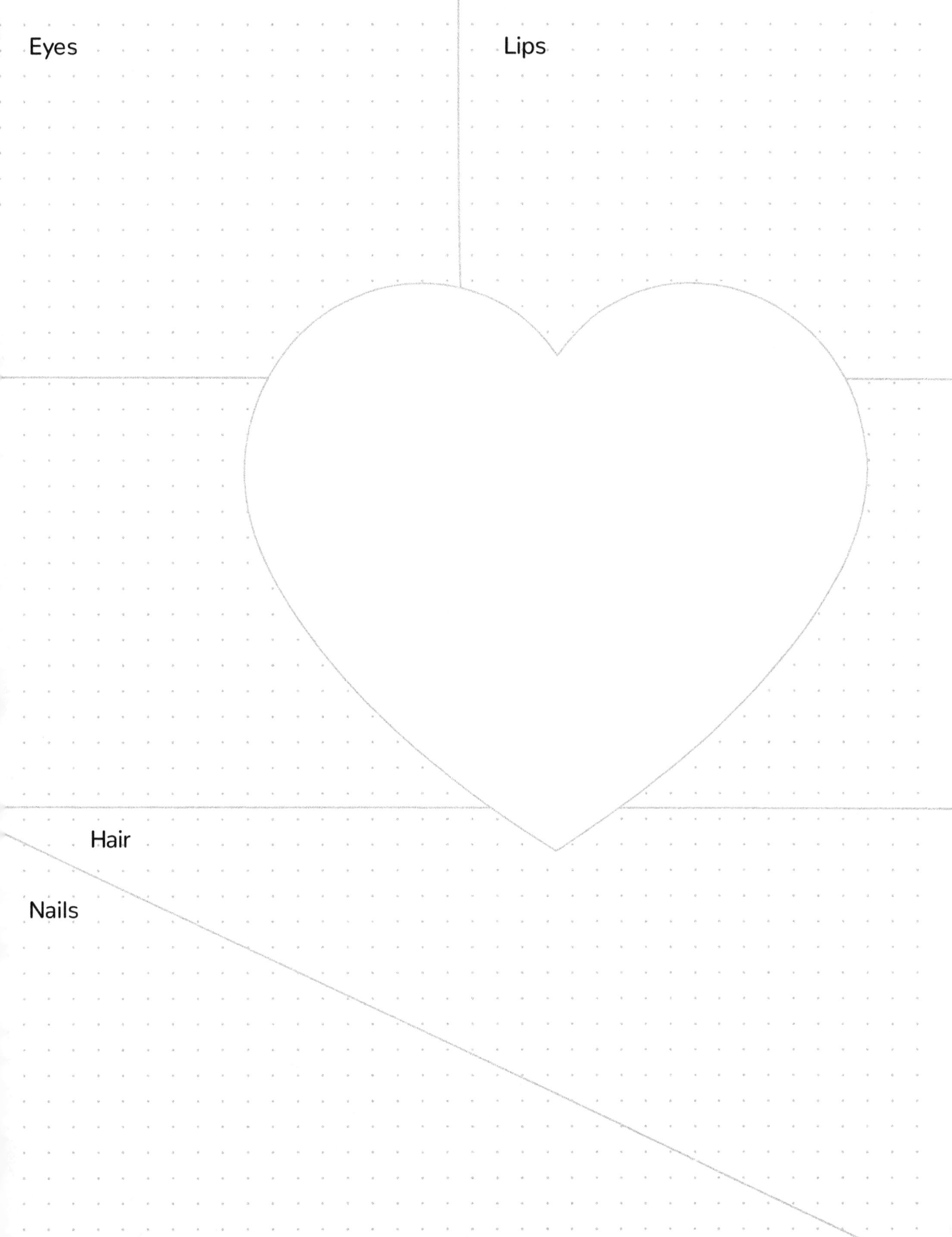
Eyes
Lips
Hair
Nails

Name of Look _________________________   Evening ○   Daytime ○

Theme ____

Face

Moisturizer

Concealer

Foundation

Highlight/Blush

Eyes

Brows

Eyelid

Liner

Crease

Mascara

Lips

Liner

Lip Color

Gloss

Notes

Makeup

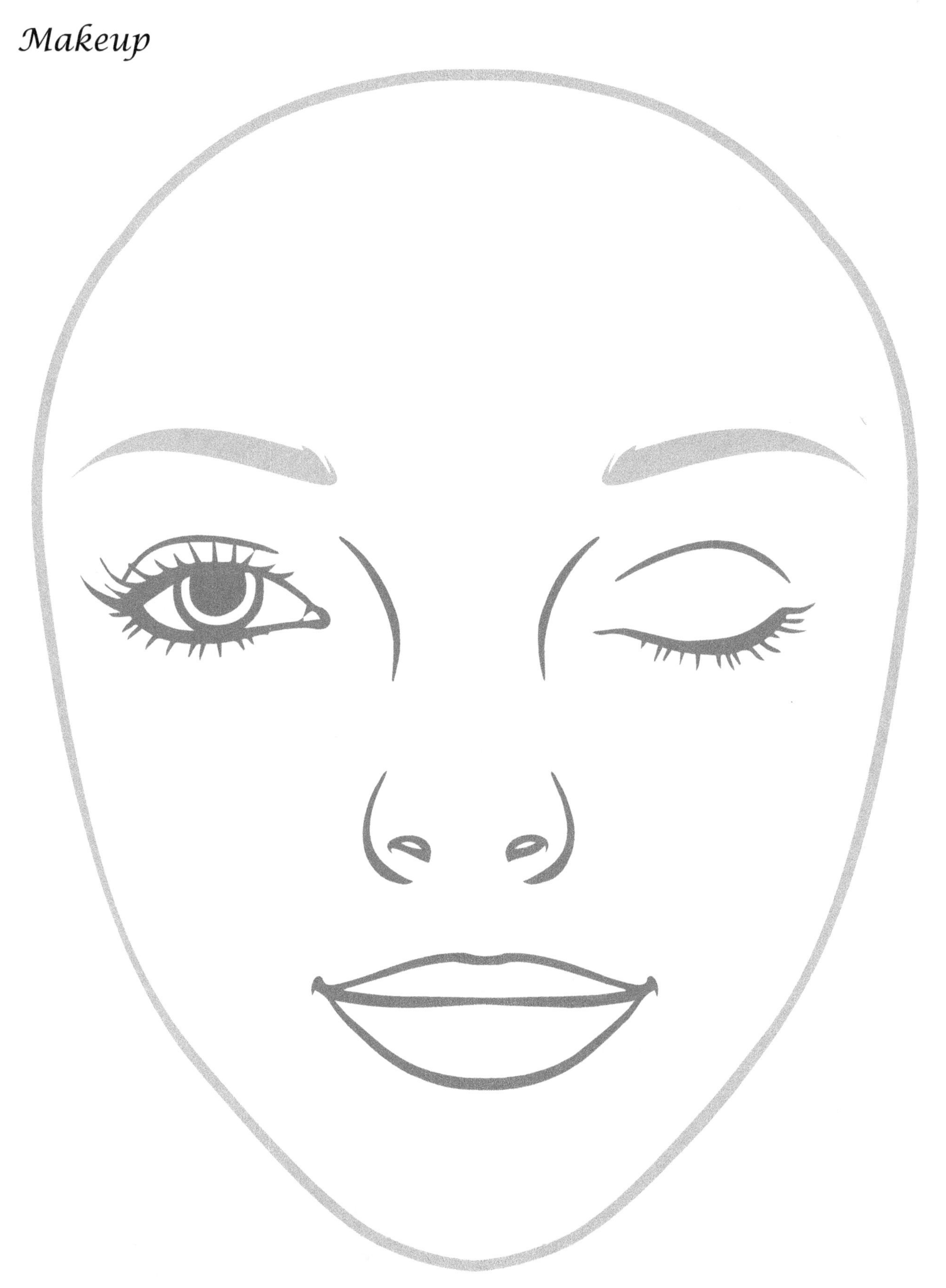

Name of Look _______________________________   **Evening** ◯   **Daytime** ◯

Theme _______________________________

Face

Moisturizer

____

Concealer

____

Foundation

____

Highlight/Blush

____

Eyes

Brows

____

Eyelid

____

Liner

____

Crease

____

Mascara

____

Lips

Liner

____

Lip Color

____

Gloss

____

____

____

Notes

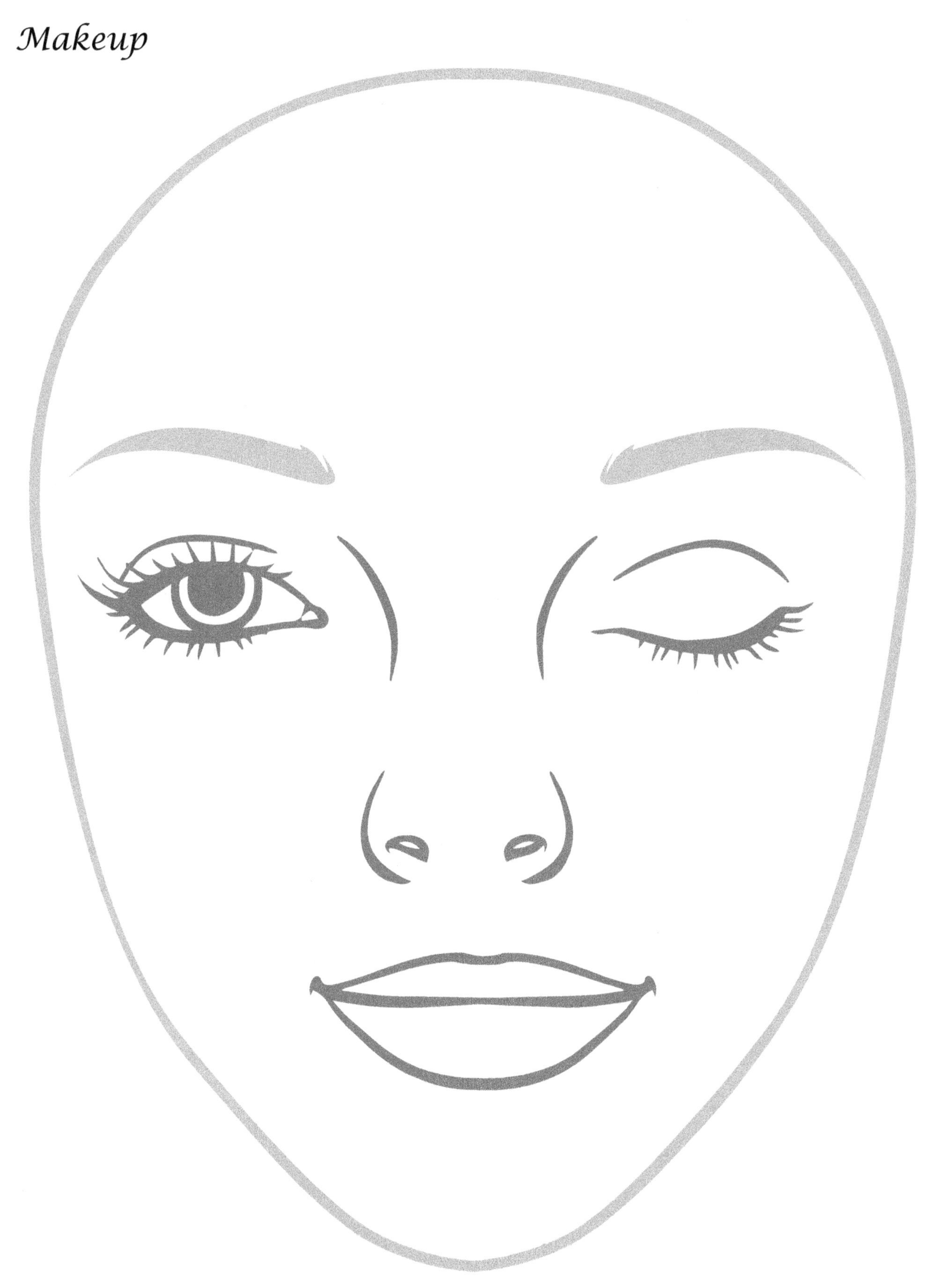

Name of Look ______________________________   Evening ◯   Daytime ◯

Theme ____

Face

Moisturizer

Concealer

Foundation

Highlight/Blush

Eyes

Brows

Eyelid

Liner

Crease

Mascara

Lips

Liner

Lip Color

Gloss

Notes

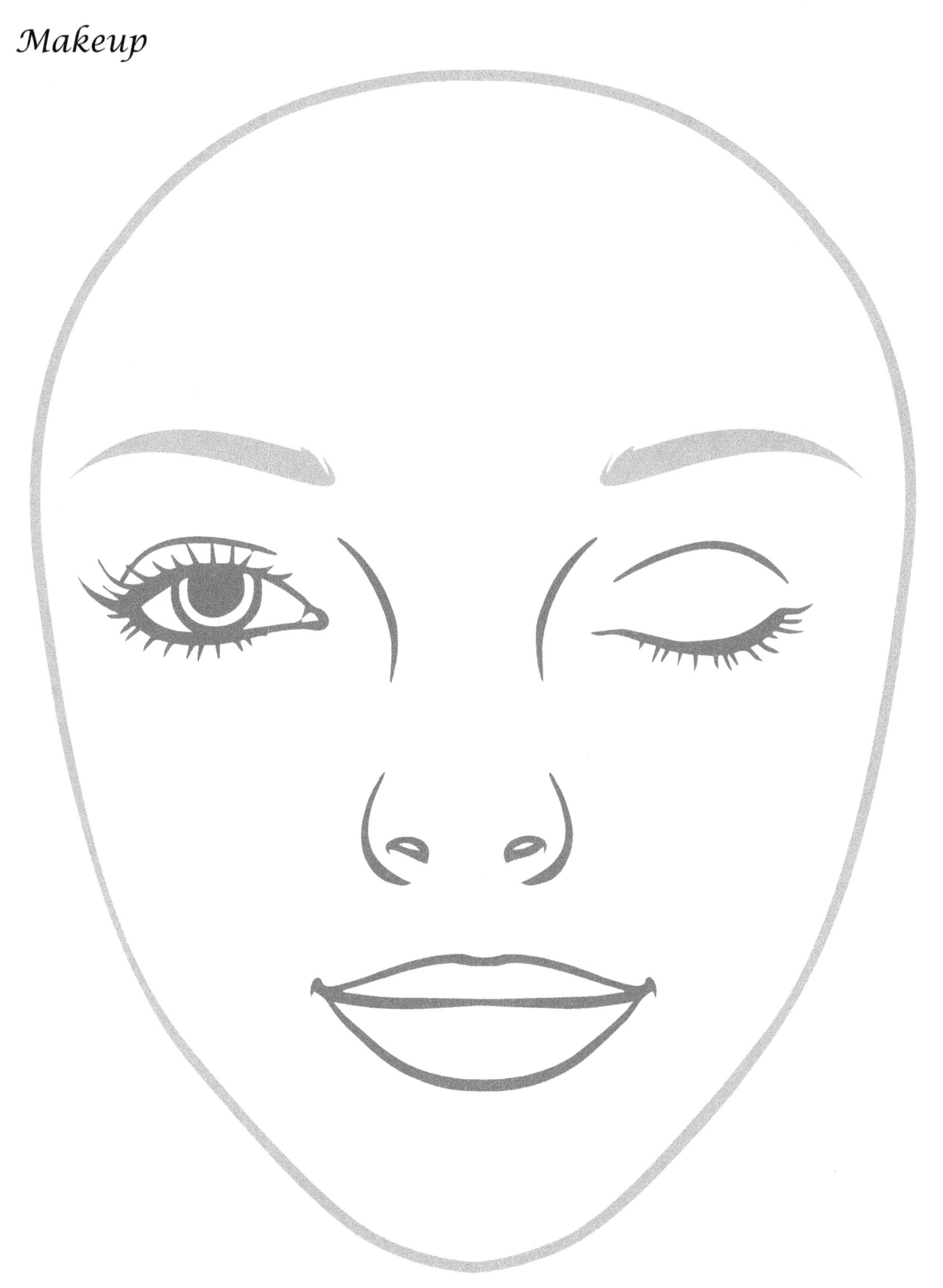
Makeup

Name of Look ______________________   **Evening** ◯   **Daytime** ◯

Theme ______________________

Face	**Eyes**	**Lips**
Moisturizer	Brows	Liner
Concealer	Eyelid	Lip Color
Foundation	Liner	Gloss
Highlight/Blush	Crease	
	Mascara	

Notes

Makeup

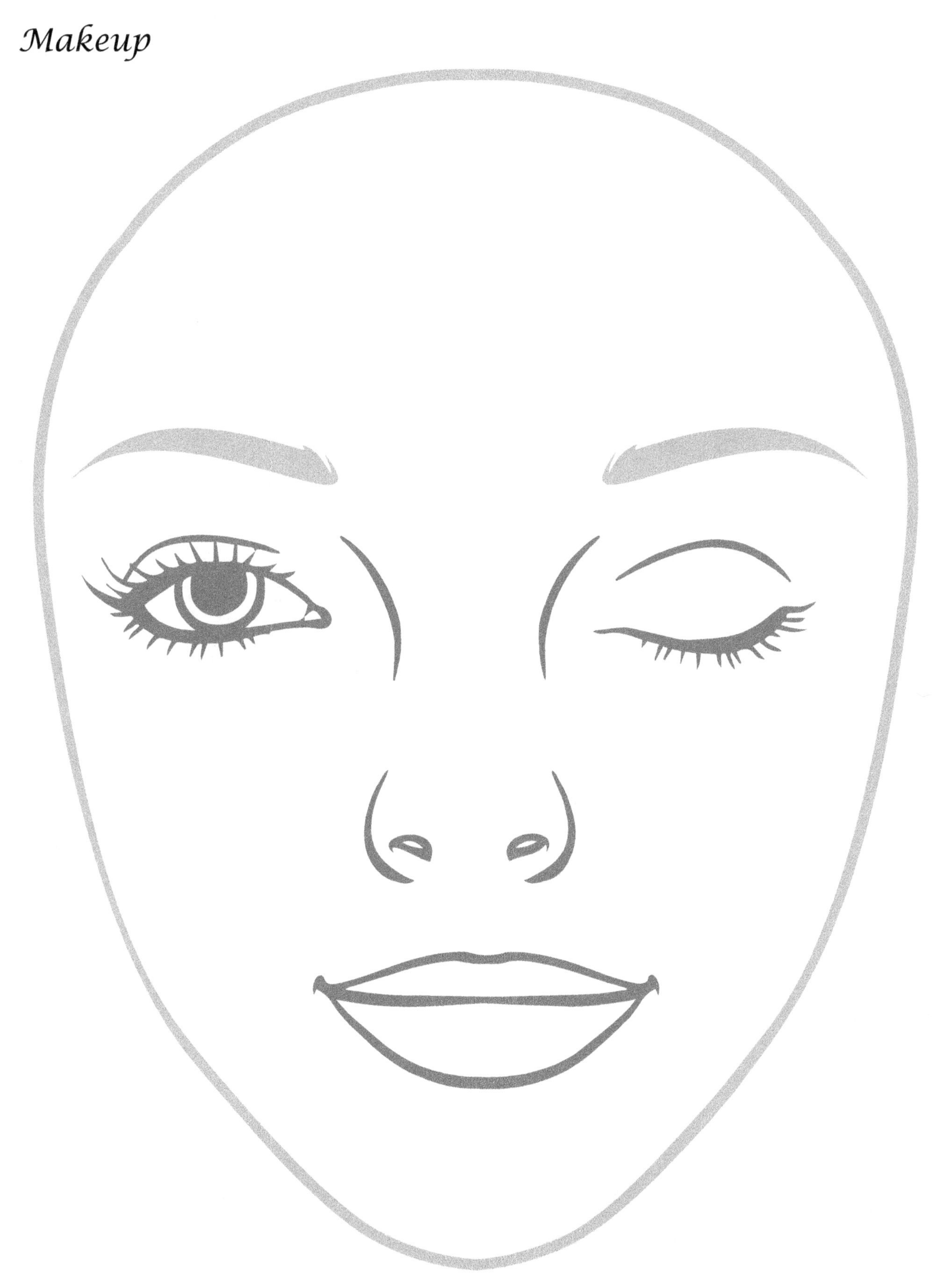

Inspiration Board Themes

Color Palettes & Patterns

Masks

Beads & Bling

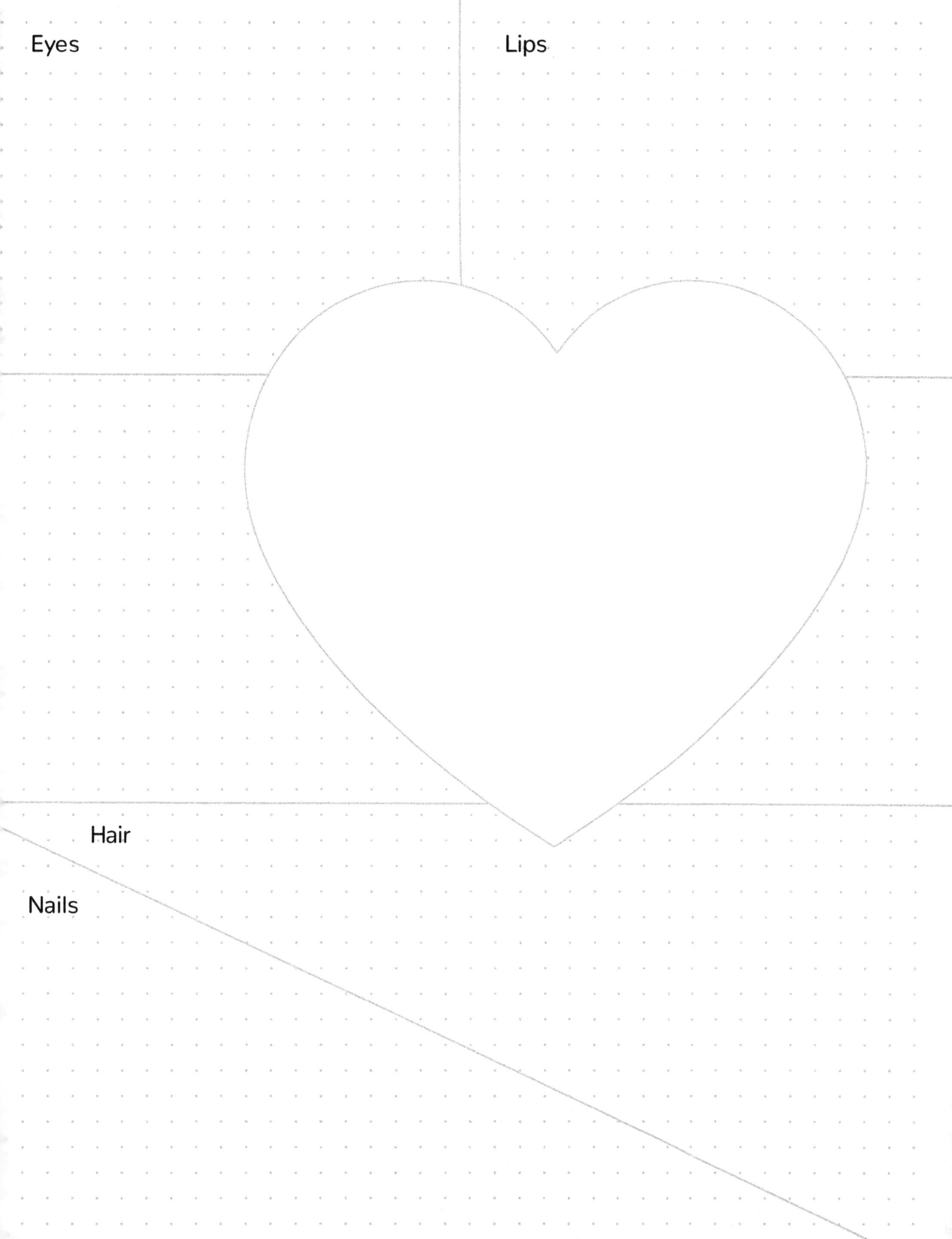
Eyes
Lips
Hair
Nails

Name of Look _______________________   **Evening** ◯   **Daytime** ◯

Theme _______________________

Face	**Eyes**	**Lips**
Moisturizer	Brows	Liner
Concealer	Eyelid	Lip Color
Foundation	Liner	Gloss
Highlight/Blush	Crease	
	Mascara	

Notes

Makeup

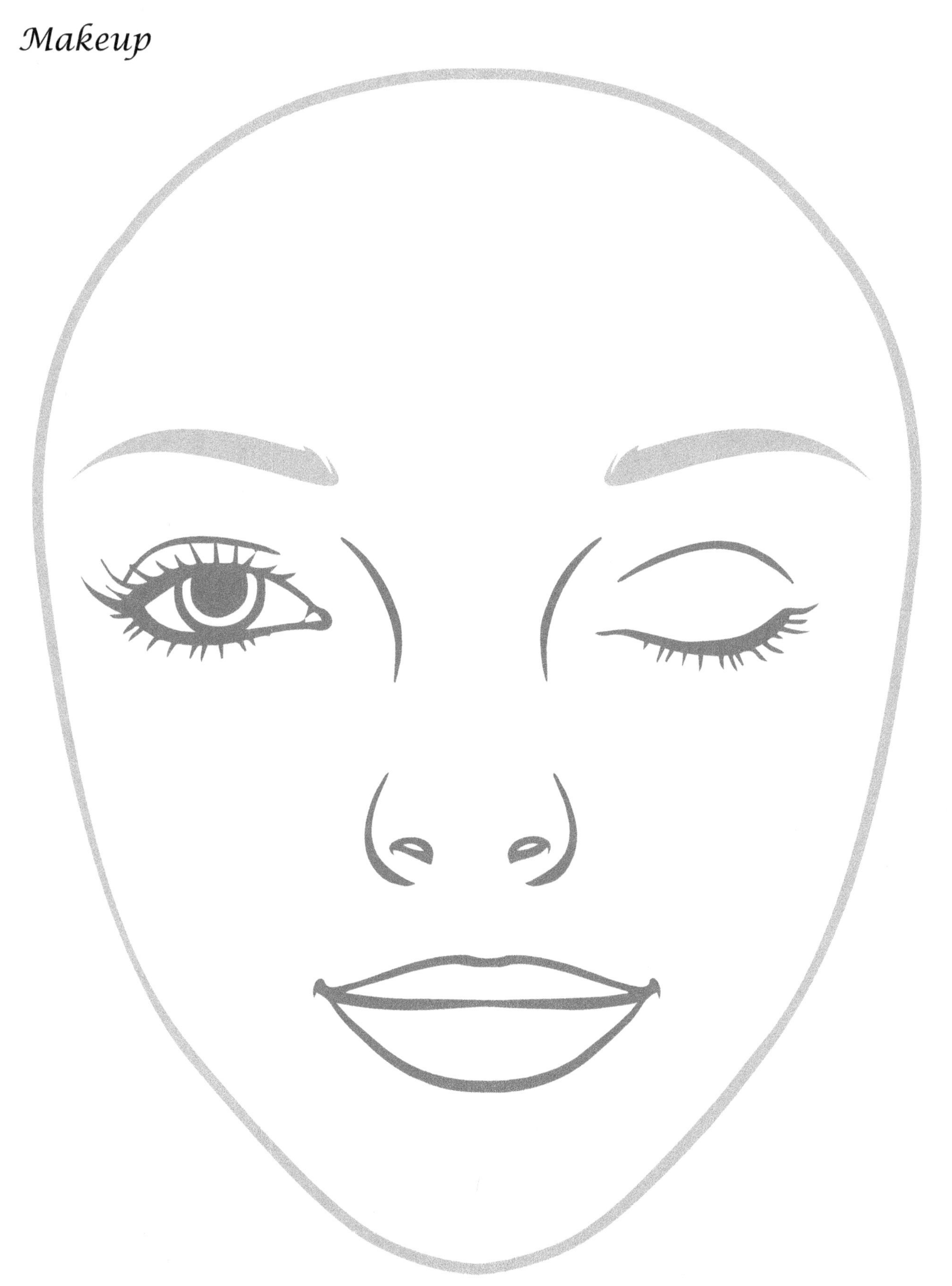

Name of Look ___________________________ Evening ◯   Daytime ◯

Theme ____

Face

Moisturizer

____

Concealer

____

Foundation

____

Highlight/Blush

____

Eyes

Brows

____

Eyelid

____

Liner

____

Crease

____

Mascara

____

Lips

Liner

____

Lip Color

____

Gloss

____

____

Notes

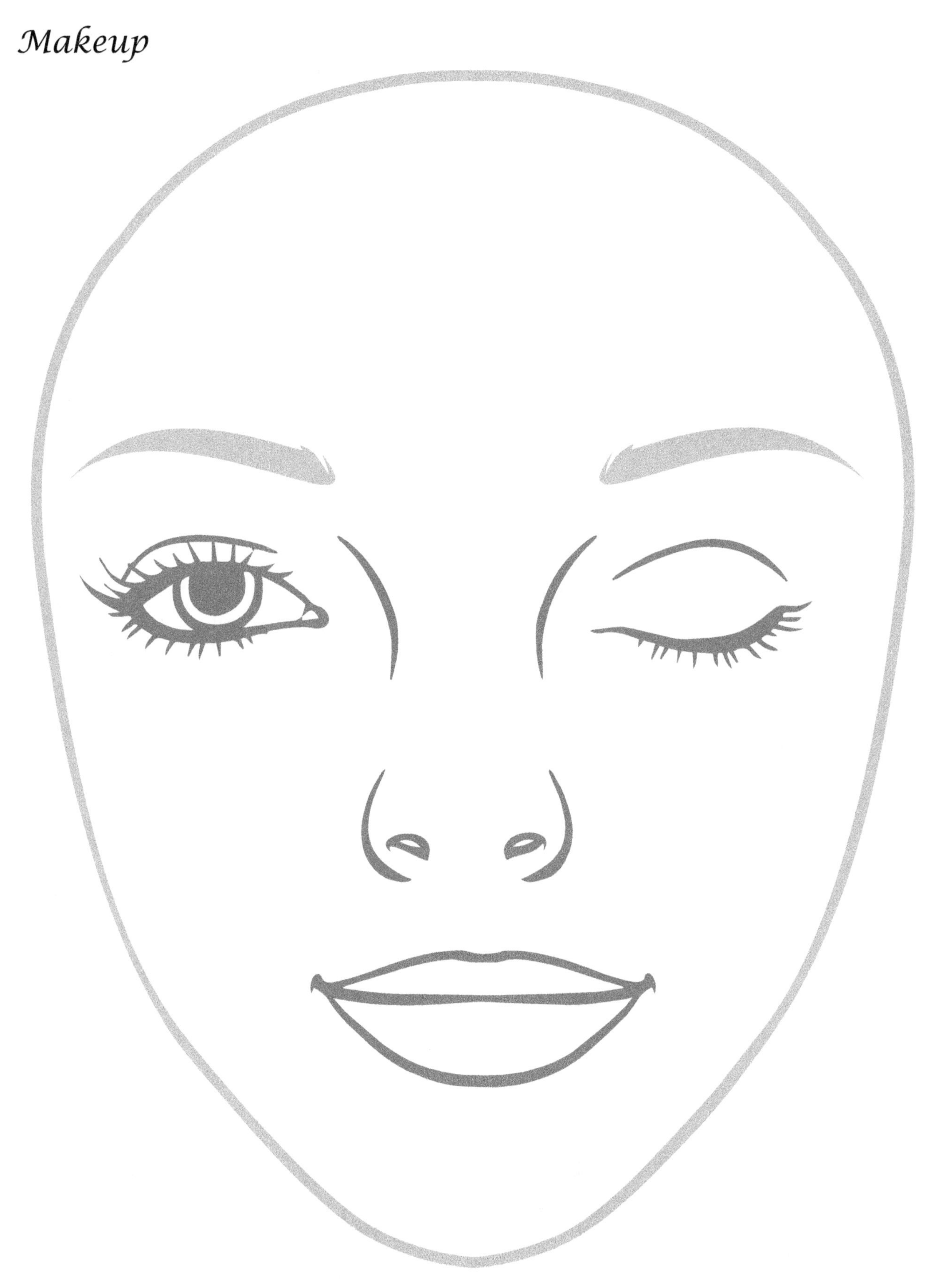

Name of Look _______________________   Evening ◯   Daytime ◯

Theme _______________________

Face

Moisturizer

____

Concealer

____

Foundation

____

Highlight/Blush

____

Eyes

Brows

____

Eyelid

____

Liner

____

Crease

____

Mascara

____

Lips

Liner

____

Lip Color

____

Gloss

____

____

____

Notes

Makeup

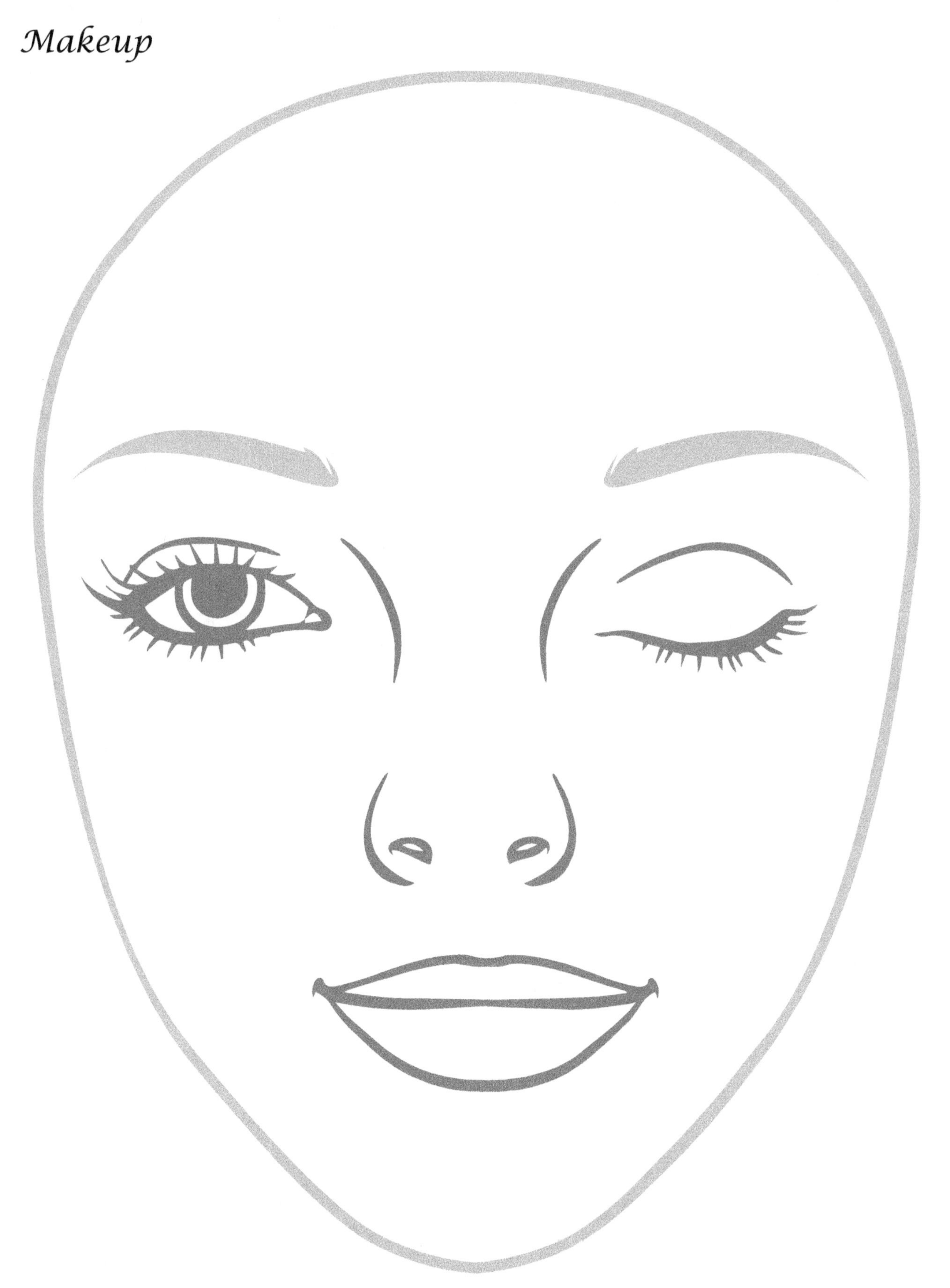

Name of Look _______________________________ Evening ○   Daytime ○

Theme ____

Face

Moisturizer

____

Concealer

____

Foundation

____

Highlight/Blush

____

Eyes

Brows

____

Eyelid

____

Liner

____

Crease

____

Mascara

____

Lips

Liner

____

Lip Color

____

Gloss

____

Notes

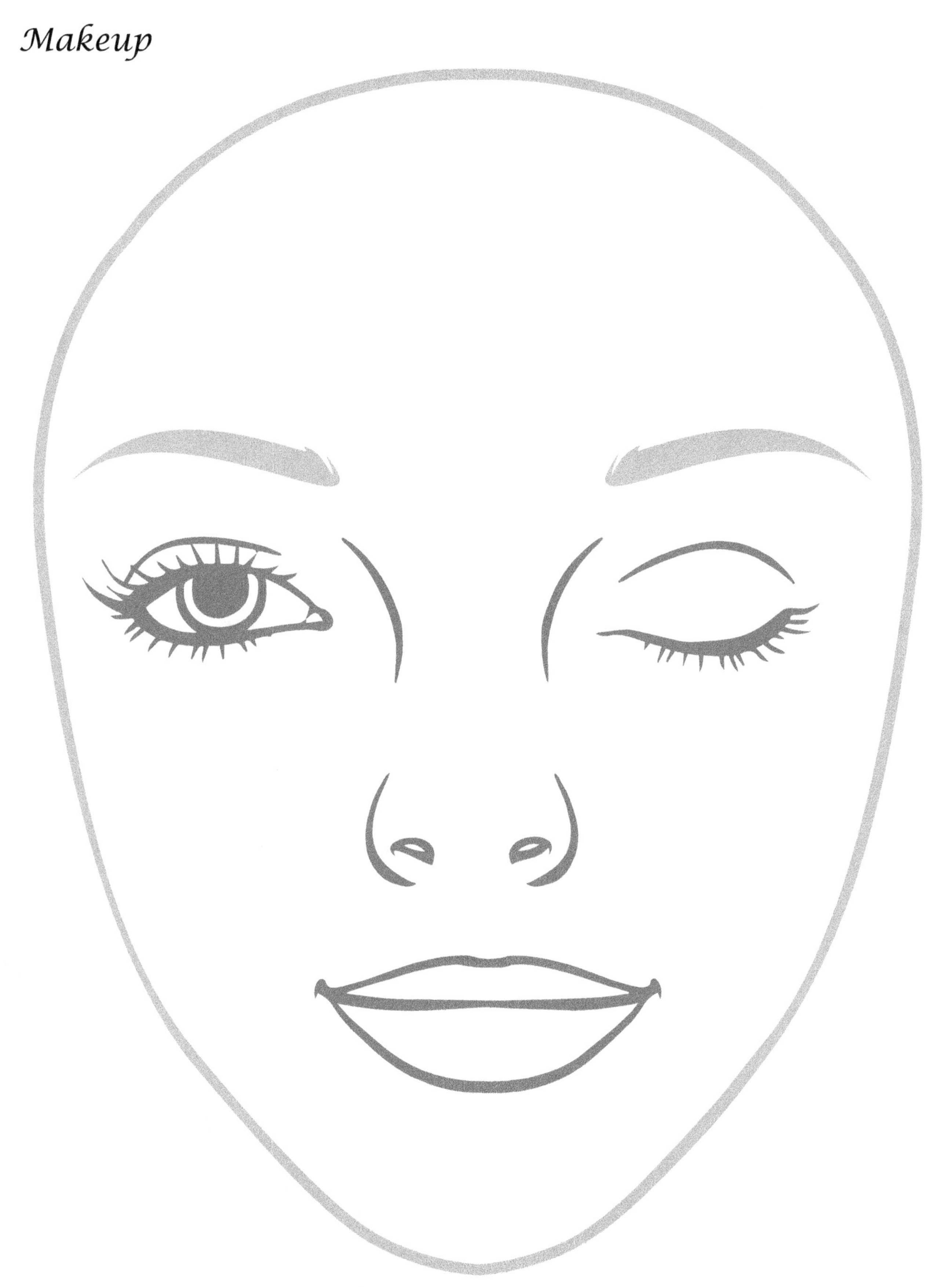

Inspiration Board

Color Palettes & Patterns

Masks

Beads & Bling

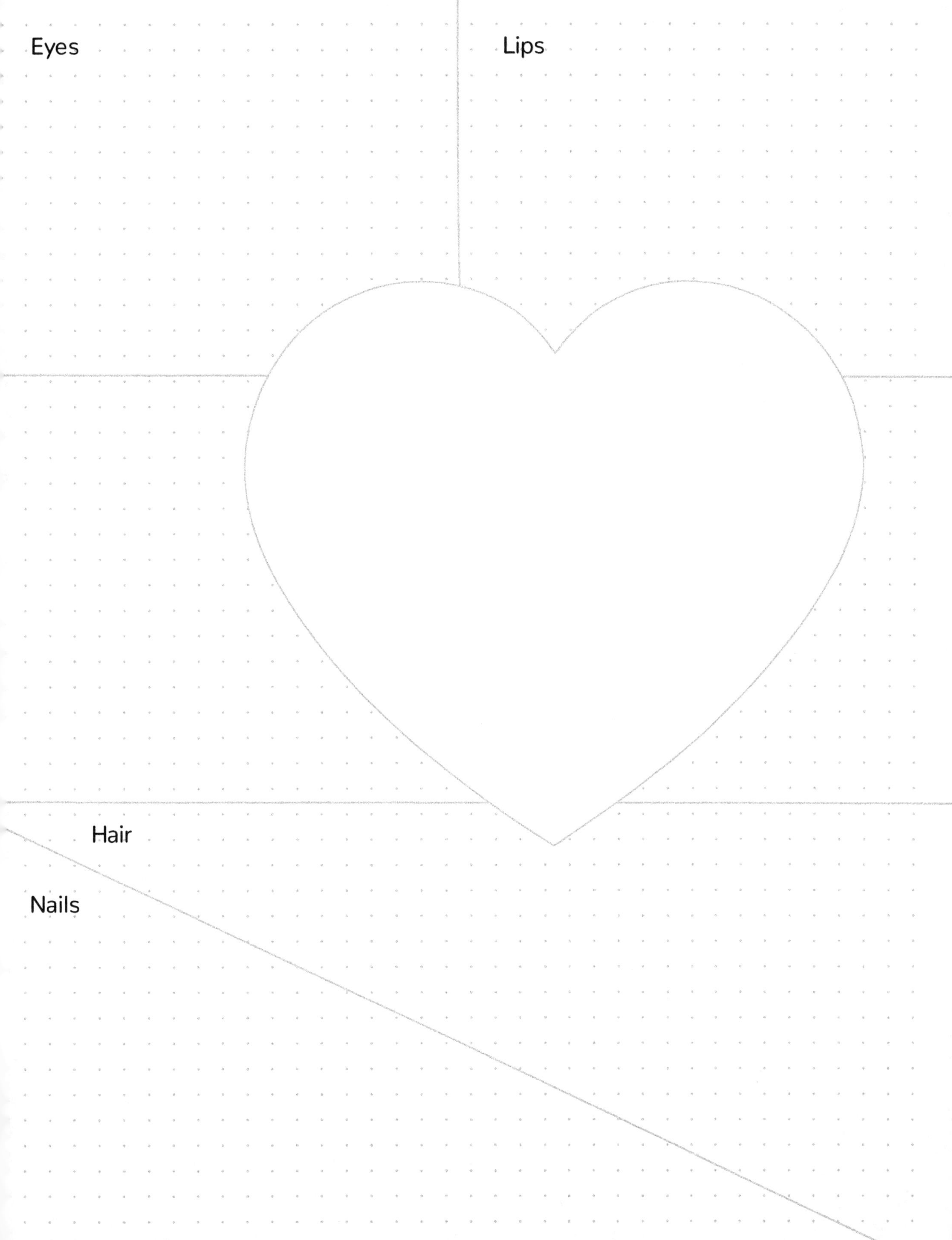

Eyes
Lips
Hair
Nails

Name of Look ______________________________   **Evening** ◯   **Daytime** ◯

Theme ______________________________

Face	**Eyes**	**Lips**
Moisturizer	Brows	Liner
Concealer	Eyelid	Lip Color
Foundation	Liner	Gloss
Highlight/Blush	Crease	
	Mascara	

Notes

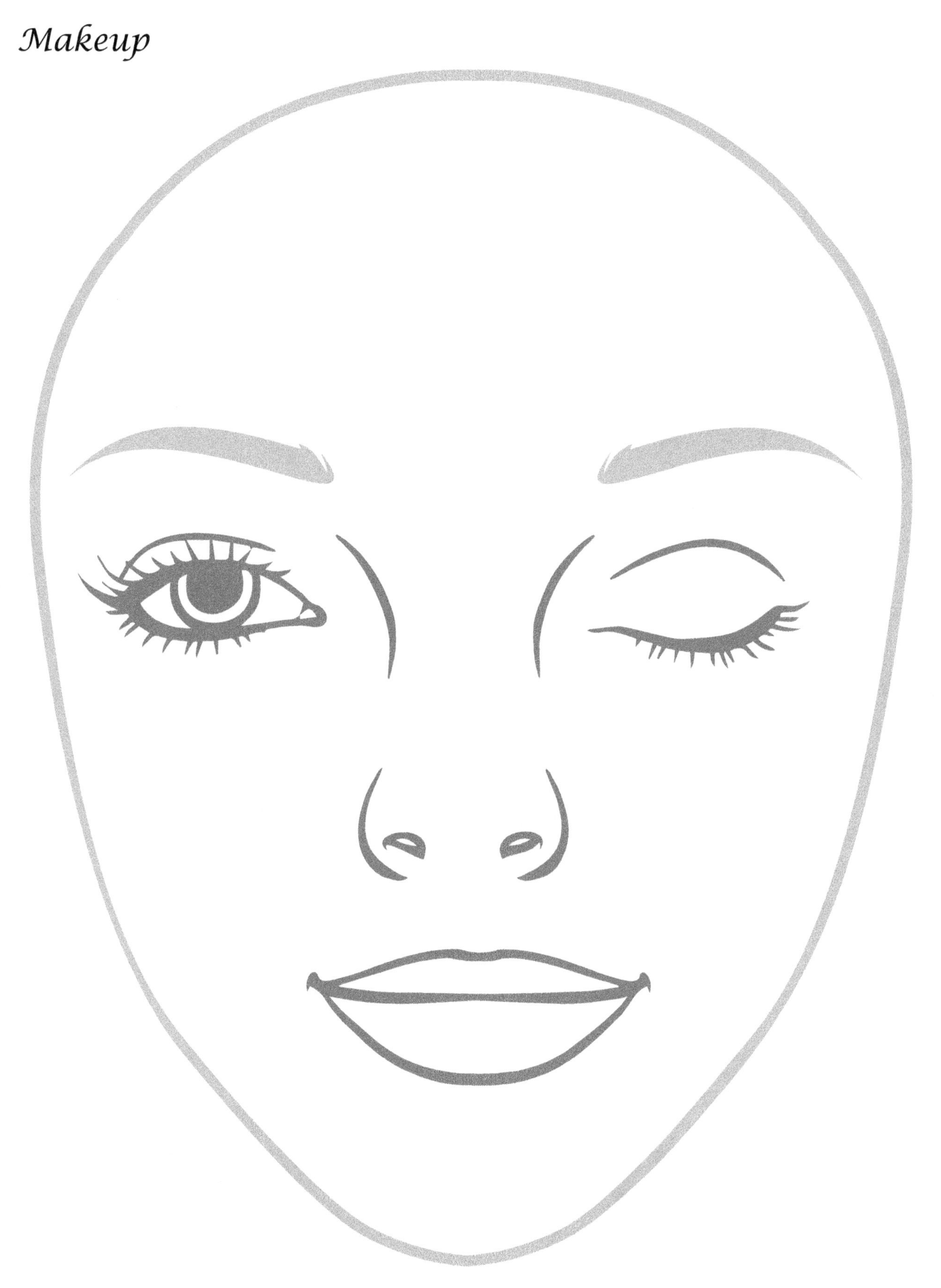
Makeup

Name of Look _______________________________   Evening ◯   Daytime ◯

Theme ____

Face

Moisturizer

Concealer

Foundation

Highlight/Blush

Eyes

Brows

Eyelid

Liner

Crease

Mascara

Lips

Liner

Lip Color

Gloss

Notes

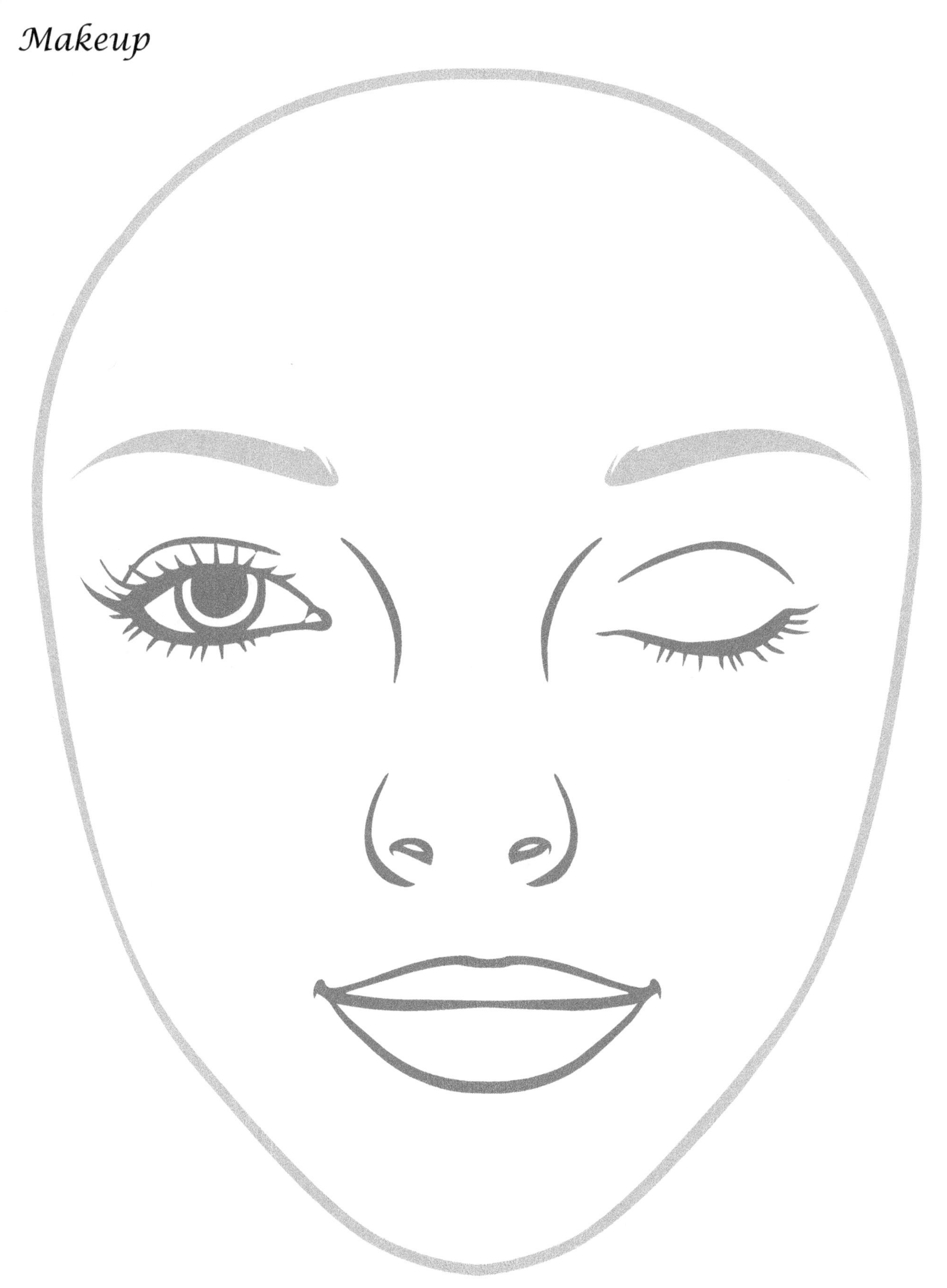

Name of Look ______________________________ **Evening** ◯   **Daytime** ◯

Theme ______________________________

Face	**Eyes**	**Lips**
Moisturizer	Brows	Liner
Concealer	Eyelid	Lip Color
Foundation	Liner	Gloss
Highlight/Blush	Crease	
	Mascara	

Notes

Makeup

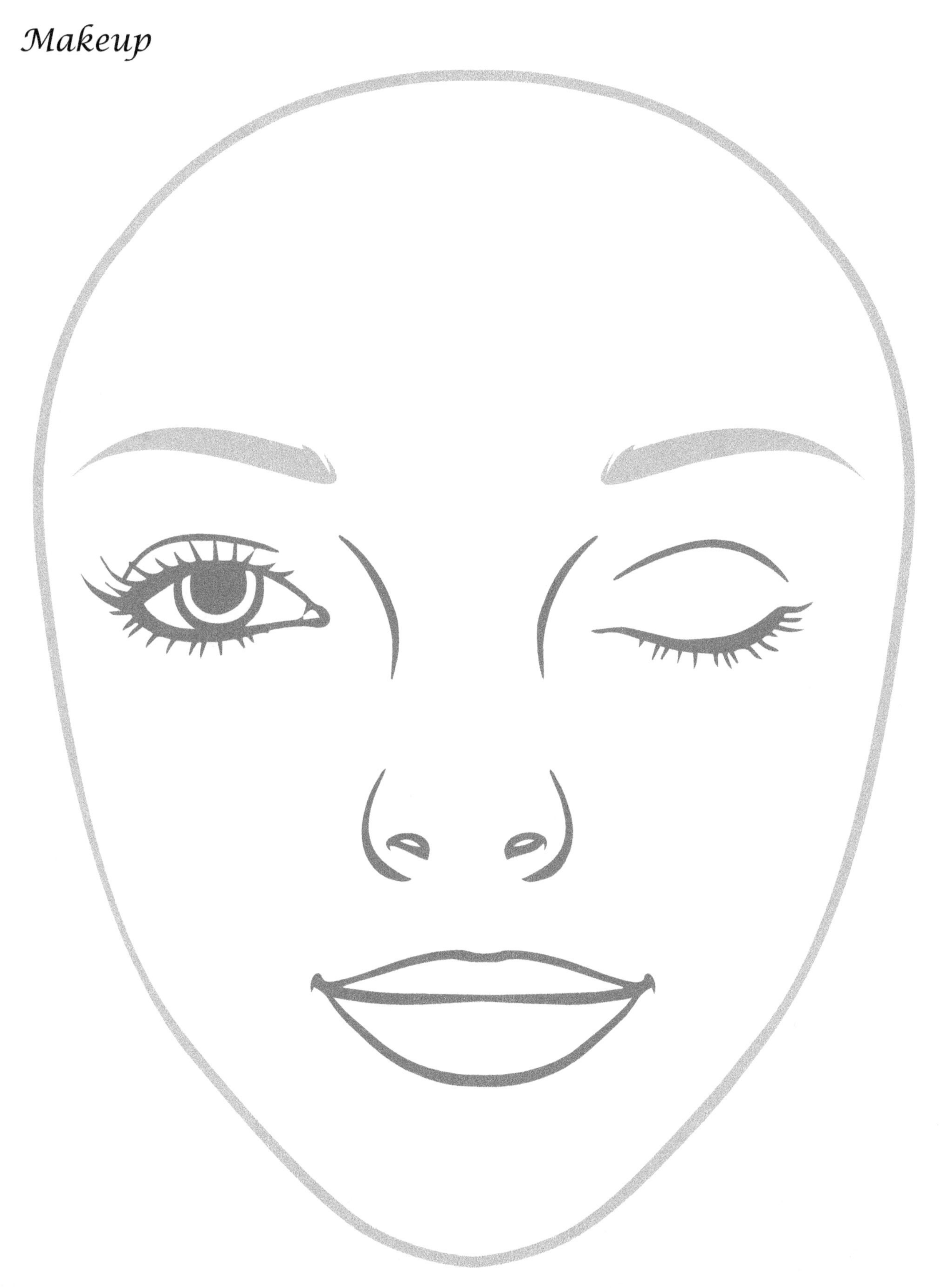

Name of Look _______________________ Evening ◯ Daytime ◯

Theme ____

Face

Moisturizer

____

Concealer

____

Foundation

____

Highlight/Blush

____

Eyes

Brows

____

Eyelid

____

Liner

____

Crease

____

Mascara

____

Lips

Liner

____

Lip Color

____

Gloss

____

Notes

Makeup

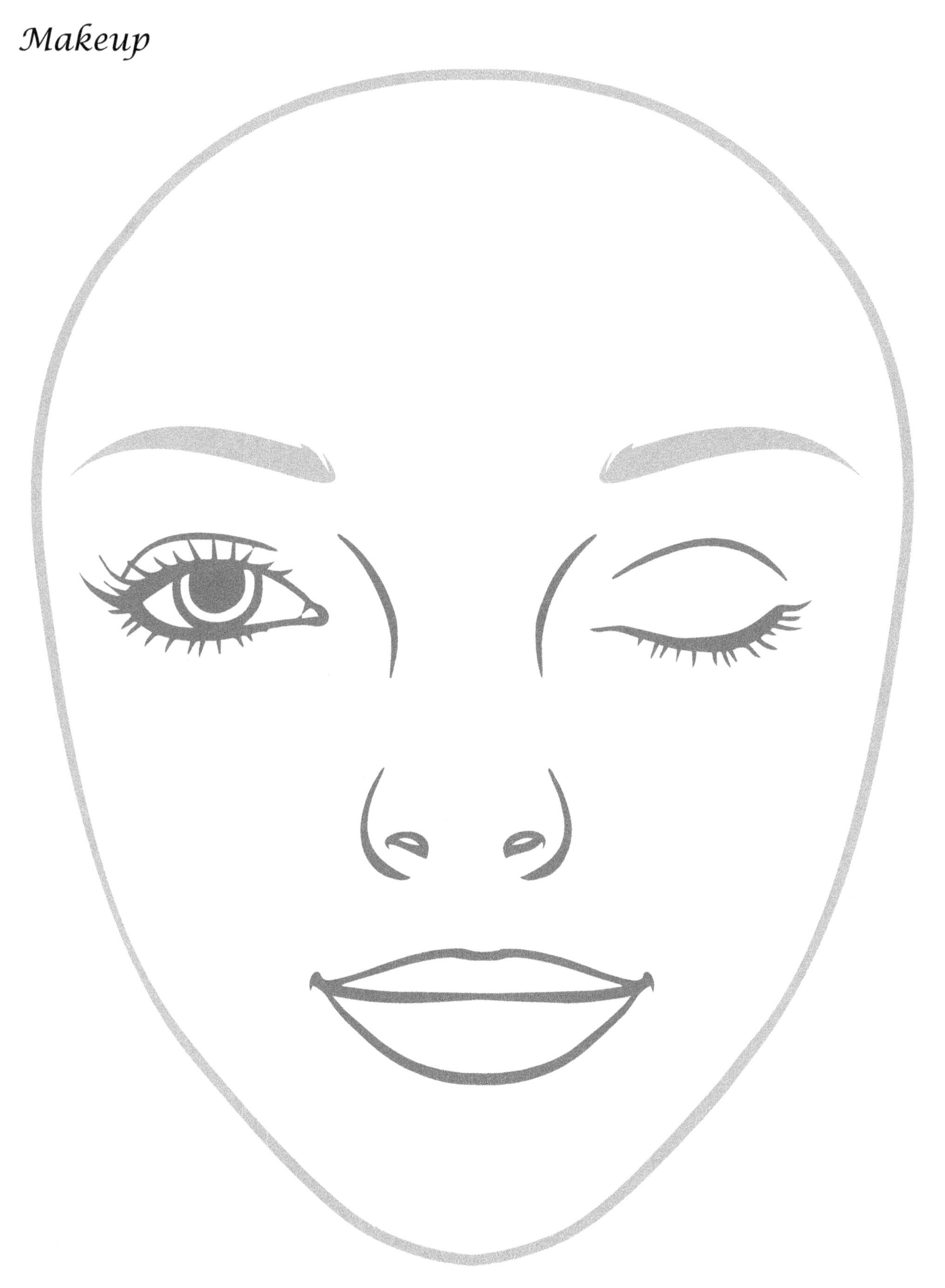

Checklist

Checklist

Checklist

Checklist

Checklist

- [ ] ......
- [ ] ......
- [ ] ......
- [ ] ......
- [ ] ......
- [ ] ......
- [ ] ......
- [ ] ......
- [ ] ......
- [ ] ......
- [ ] ......
- [ ] ......
- [ ] ......
- [ ] ......
- [ ] ......
- [ ] ......
- [ ] ......
- [ ] ......
- [ ] ......

Checklist

Checklist

www.ingramcontent.com/pod-product-compliance
Lightning Source LLC
Chambersburg PA
CBHW081620250726
48657CB00009B/2651